CHAIR YOGA FOR SENIORS OVER 60

Easy Step by step Guide for Seniors to Build Strength with Low impact Exercise, increase balance and Improve Flexibility With Ease

Glenn M. Howard

TABLE OF CONTENT

INTRODUCTION

In terms of fitness and well-being, chair yoga stands out as a gentle yet very effective practice designed exclusively for seniors over the age of 60.

As people age, maintaining physical fitness becomes increasingly important, and chair yoga offers an accessible way to promote total well-being. This type of yoga is very good for seniors who may have mobility issues or desire a more gentle fitness program.

Chair yoga combines classic yoga postures with the support of a chair, making it a versatile and inclusive practice. Seniors may easily incorporate chair yoga into their daily routines, reaping a variety of benefits that go beyond flexibility and balance.

One of the key benefits is the relief of frequent aging-related bodily aches and pains. Chair yoga's mild stretches and exercises improve flexibility, promote joint health, and relieve pain.

Furthermore, chair yoga improves cardiovascular health, which is an important component of overall fitness for seniors.

Seniors who engage in regulated and focused movements can improve blood circulation, reduce blood pressure, and strengthen their cardiovascular systems.

Chair yoga's versatility makes it an excellent alternative for people wishing to enhance their cardiovascular health without indulging in hard exercises.

Weight control is another area where chair yoga demonstrates its effectiveness for seniors. Despite the restricted mobility that may come with aging, chair yoga offers a way to engage in physical exercise that promotes weight reduction.

Strength-building workouts and regulated motions can help to improve body composition.One of the primary benefits of chair yoga for seniors is the time savings it provides.

Seniors may easily include chair yoga into their regular schedules because the practices are shorter in duration. This time-saving feature promotes consistency, which is essential for maximizing the benefits of any workout plan.

Chair yoga appears as a complete option for adults over 60, providing a way to avoid body pains, improve cardiovascular health, and efficiently control weight.

Its versatility and time efficiency make it an important addition to the lives of seniors, encouraging not just physical well-being but also a sense of calm and awareness.

Chapter 1: Unveiling the Healing Power of Seated Wellness

In the holistic well-being of seniors over 60, the transforming practice of seated health takes center stage, particularly via the soft embrace of chair yoga.

This sitting modality effortlessly integrates therapeutic movements with mindfulness, providing a customized approach to promoting physical, mental, and emotional balance.

Seniors can go on a rejuvenating adventure by immersing themselves in the tranquil world of seated wellness. Controlled postures and regular breathing work together to develop flexibility while also improving circulation, which is essential for general health. Seniors can enjoy a restored sense of vigor by engaging in intentional movements, offsetting the effects of sedentary behavior.

Furthermore, seated health, such as chair yoga, offers a source of comfort for persons dealing with physical restrictions.

Tailored sequences guarantee that people with different levels of mobility may participate in the therapeutic dance of stretching and relaxation.

This openness develops a sense of camaraderie and confidence, eliminating the myth that age should limit one's physical ability.

Aside from the physical benefits, sitting wellness has a positive impact on mental and emotional health. Chair yoga reduces stress and promotes a serene state of mind.

Mindfulness, a key component of this practice, allows seniors to connect with the present moment, cultivating resilience and tranquility in the face of life's adversities.

In essence, chair yoga for seniors over 60 reveals a powerful route for comprehensive health. It goes beyond the traditional limitations of physical exercise, providing a holistic approach that addresses the various aspects of well-being.
Seniors may experience the transformational power of seated wellbeing by gently embracing the

harmonious connection of mind, body, and spirit.

Connecting Mind and Body through Chair Yoga

Chair yoga is a relaxing exercise that integrates the mind and body. This moderate type of yoga allows conventional postures to be practiced while sitting, making it more accessible and useful to people with limited mobility.

Chair yoga promotes overall well-being by combining breath and movement.
Chair yoga allows seniors to improve flexibility, strength, and balance.

The practice emphasizes purposeful, controlled movements, developing a stronger connection between the body and the mind.
As elders smoothly shift from one posture to the next, the emphasis on

mindfulness promotes a keen awareness of each delicate feeling.

The combination of breathwork and mild stretches in chair yoga has therapeutic benefits for elders. Deep, deliberate breathing brings oxygen into the body, producing calm and mental clarity.

The relaxing effects of regulated breathing complement the physical advantages, giving a comprehensive approach to wellbeing.

Furthermore, chair yoga is an effective stress-reduction technique. Seniors move through a series of sitting positions, releasing tension and generating a sense of relaxation. The mind becomes more attentive to the present moment, forming a mental sanctuary in which external problems might momentarily disappear.

Chair yoga's adjustability makes it a welcoming and accessible practice. Seniors may adjust the difficulty of the postures to meet their own requirements, instilling a sense of empowerment.

The addition of mindfulness and breath awareness transforms this kind of yoga into not only a physical workout but also a contemplative journey, providing a sanctuary where the mind and body intersect for improved overall well-being.

In essence, chair yoga for seniors over 60 connects the physical and mental domains, creating a loving environment for self-care and renewal.

This practice becomes a conduit for holistic health by including conscious movement and breath, generating a profound connection between the mind and body.

Embarking on a Journey of Senior Serenity

Beginning a journey of senior peace entails adopting holistic health techniques targeted for those aged 60 and up.

Chair yoga emerges as a gentle yet transforming way for seniors to improve their physical, mental, and emotional health.

This approachable style of yoga caters to the specific requirements of older people, encouraging flexibility, balance, and relaxation without the need for difficult poses.

In the area of senior tranquility, chair yoga shines as a light of inclusion. Seniors sit comfortably in recliners and do a sequence of modified yoga poses tailored to their mobility and comfort. These exercises are intended to increase joint flexibility and muscular strength, promoting a sensation of renewal.

The regular flow of chair yoga enables elders to practice mindful breathing, which reduces tension and promotes a calm mental state.

Chair yoga has a significant impact on emotional resilience in addition to its physical advantages. Seniors feel a profound sense of calm as they link breath and movement, developing mind-body balance.

This contemplative feature of chair yoga acts as a pathway to inner peace, allowing elders to face the obstacles of aging with grace and calm.

Furthermore, the social nature of chair yoga courses adds to the overall feeling of senior peace.

Participants create a supportive community by sharing their experiences and encouraging one another.

This companionship creates a pleasant environment, promoting the notion that age is no limit to personal development and well-being.

Beginning a path of senior peace with chair yoga provides a balanced combination of physical, mental, and emotional advantages.

Seniors over the age of 60 can improve their well-being by embracing this peaceful practice, which fosters a comprehensive feeling of tranquility that transcends the restrictions that come with aging.

Chapter 2: Understanding the Aging Body

As our bodies gracefully age, it is critical to adopt routines that address our changing physical demands.

Chair yoga emerges as a gentle yet effective alternative for seniors over 60, offering a comprehensive approach to preserving health and well-being.

Understanding the aging body is critical for designing training regimens, and chair yoga effectively tackles the particular obstacles that seniors confront.

The aging process affects flexibility, balance, and strength. Chair yoga acknowledges these changes by providing modified postures that may be practiced easily while seated or with the chair for support. This adaptation allows elders to engage in mindful meditation without placing undue strain on joints or muscles.

One noticeable characteristic of chair yoga is its emphasis on flexibility. Gentle stretches and motions target specific regions, increasing joint mobility and reducing stiffness.

This not only improves physical comfort but also increases total flexibility, making daily chores easier for elders.

Chair yoga also focuses on balance. The danger of falling rises as we age, and practicing balance-centric postures while seated on a chair gives a solid foundation.

Seniors may improve and maintain their balance without jeopardizing their safety, instilling confidence in their actions.

Chair yoga also focuses on strengthening muscles that are necessary for daily activities. Seniors can gain and retain muscle mass by carefully selecting positions, resulting in better stability and functionality.

This feature of the technique is very effective for reducing muscle mass loss, which is often connected with aging.

Incorporating chair yoga into the routines of adults over 60 has more than just physical advantages. It promotes awareness and relaxation, hence improving mental health.

Breathing exercises and meditation, perfectly blended into chair yoga, create a serene environment for seniors to reconnect with their bodies and build a sense of inner calm.

Chair yoga for seniors over 60 is a deliberate reaction to the changes that come with aging.

It recognizes the intricacies of the aging body and provides a personalized approach that improves flexibility, balance, and strength while improving general well-being.

The practice is more than simply an exercise program; it is a comprehensive path toward a better, more mindful lifestyle.

Navigating the Landscape of Senior Health

In the world of senior wellness, investigating multiple paths for well-being becomes critical, and one such path gaining popularity is chair yoga designed for people over the age of 60.

Chair yoga is a comprehensive approach to physical and mental wellness, providing a gentle yet effective way to negotiate the particular landscape of senior well-being.

The practice includes modified yoga positions that can be performed while seated, giving elders an accessible and safe way to stay active.

Gentle stretches and controlled movements not only enhance flexibility but also help to preserve joint health, which is especially important for seniors dealing with the problems of aging.

Chair yoga goes beyond the traditional definition of physical exercise by including mindfulness and stress reduction techniques.

Breathwork and meditation help elders achieve mental clarity and relaxation, which promotes emotional well-being.

In an era of constant stress, these characteristics of chair yoga become vital skills for negotiating the often complex landscape of senior care.

Furthermore, the social component of chair yoga lessons must be considered. Seniors develop a feeling of community and companionship, building ties that are beneficial to their mental health.

The group energy of a chair yoga class fosters an inclusive environment, encouraging a shared journey to wellbeing.

As we traverse the terrain of elder health, chair yoga stands out as a model of adaptation and inclusiveness.

Its delicate yet strong influence on physical, mental, and social well-being highlights its importance in meeting the special requirements of seniors over 60.

By embracing this holistic practice, elders may start on a journey that not only improves their physical vigor but also fosters a deep feeling of inner balance and camaraderie.

Crafting Chair Yoga Solutions for Aging Bodies

Crafting solutions for aging bodies through chair yoga provides adults over the age of 60 with a personalized approach to improving their health.

This sitting exercise allows people to easily incorporate moderate movements, stretches, and breathwork into their routine. The major focus is on increasing flexibility, strength, and relaxation while sitting comfortably in a chair.

One significant advantage of chair yoga for elders is its versatility. The practice accommodates a wide range of fitness levels and physical abilities, making it accessible to a large number of people.

Seniors can benefit from a low-impact workout that enhances joint health and decreases stiffness by using carefully chosen positions.

This personalized approach addresses the particular demands of aging bodies, allowing participants to continue an active lifestyle while avoiding undue strain.

Chair yoga also emphasizes breath awareness, which promotes mindfulness and reduces stress. Controlled breathing can help seniors relax, improve their mental health, and increase their resilience to daily challenges.

This comprehensive approach treats both the physical and mental elements of aging, resulting in a greater sense of vitality.

Incorporating props like straps and blocks into chair yoga also allows for a more in-depth examination of postures and a wider range of motion.

Seniors can steadily improve their practice, increasing strength and flexibility over time.

The inclusive nature of chair yoga creates a supportive environment for elders, fostering social interaction and a shared commitment to well-being.

Chair yoga for seniors over 60 provides a mindful and adaptive way to assist aging bodies. Individuals can develop physical and mental resilience by engaging in mindful movement, breathing exercises, and the use of props.

This approach to yoga encourages variety, acknowledging and honoring seniors' individual journeys to holistic well-being.

Empowering Seniors with Yogic Wisdom

Empowering seniors with yoga wisdom, particularly via chair yoga designed for people over the age of 60, provides a transforming approach to physical and mental health.

Maintaining a healthy lifestyle becomes increasingly important as we age, and yoga's holistic principles provide seniors with a gentle yet effective way to improve their entire quality of life.

Chair yoga elegantly modifies conventional yoga positions, making them accessible to elders of all mobility abilities.

This simplified practice is done while seated or supported by a chair, allowing seniors to reap the full benefits of yoga without the need for difficult floor positions. The integration of breathwork, moderate stretches, and mindfulness practices promotes inner peace and resilience.

One of the most impressive features of chair yoga for seniors is its ability to increase flexibility and range of motion. The mild motions improve joint mobility, reduce stiffness, and relieve the pain associated with aging.

As elders engage in these modified yogic practices, they gain new strength and balance, developing a sense of confidence and independence.

Furthermore, chair yoga promotes a mind-body connection, which benefits cognitive health. Seniors are encouraged to focus on the present moment, which promotes mental clarity and emotional stability. The contemplative components of chair yoga might help with stress reduction, perhaps easing feelings of anxiety or despair that can come with age.

Social connectedness is another important aspect of seniors' well-being. Chair yoga courses create a friendly environment in which people may share their experiences and form important friendships.

This sensation of belonging boosts mental resilience and reduces feelings of loneliness.

Chair yoga for seniors goes beyond the physical sphere, providing a road to overall empowerment.

Seniors over 60 who embrace yogic teachings in a chair-based practice can manage their aging journey with increased physical energy, mental clarity, and a profound sense of community, eventually enhancing their golden years with a revived passion for life.

Chapter 3: The Art of Seated Asanas

Chair yoga for seniors over 60 combines relaxation and physical well-being via the practice of sitting asanas.

This particular type of yoga is designed to meet the specific requirements and skills of older people, encouraging a gentle yet effective approach to preserving flexibility and increasing awareness.

Seated asanas, or postures, are the cornerstone of chair yoga, allowing elderly to enjoy the practice in comfort and stability.

These postures, carefully designed for sitting positions, accommodate people with varied degrees of mobility, making them accessible to a wide range of elders.

 The art is in the seamless integration of breath control and gentle movements, which creates a holistic experience that benefits overall health.

The chair serves as a prop for support, allowing elderly to start on a journey of self-discovery and physical regeneration.

Participants can improve their flexibility, posture, and circulation by stretching mindfully and controlling their breathing.

The art of sitting asanas in chair yoga highlights the significance of tailoring conventional poses to the restrictions and comfort levels of seniors, fostering a sense of empowerment and inclusion.

Furthermore, the practice goes beyond the physical sphere, exploring the mental and emotional dimensions of well-being. Seated meditation, which is integrated into chair yoga sessions, promotes inner calm and quiet.

Seniors are taught to connect with their breath, calm their minds, and enter a meditative state, which promotes mental clarity and stress reduction.

In essence, the technique of sitting asanas in chair yoga for seniors over 60 is a comprehensive approach to health and wellness.

It embraces the integration of movement, breath, and mindfulness, providing a personalized experience that benefits the body, mind, and soul. Seniors can go on a path to better health and a deeper connection with themselves by engaging in this artistic discipline.

Embracing Tranquility: Seated Yoga Poses

In the area of holistic well-being for seniors over 60, the gentle technique of chair yoga reveals a route to serenity via sitting positions.

As seniors encounter the calming realm of chair yoga, they may embrace tranquility and embark on a rejuvenating journey.

Seated yoga positions provide a unique combination of relaxation and physical activity, promoting a peaceful connection between mind, body, and breath.

As elders glide elegantly through the series of sitting positions, the chair serves as a helpful ally, offering stability and accessibility. Each position is

designed to increase flexibility, balance, and awareness without requiring complex floor movements.
The rhythmic flow of sitting yoga promotes a soothing environment, allowing seniors to have a peaceful experience that transcends physical restrictions.

From mild twists to thoughtful stretches, the sitting yoga poses for seniors over 60 are designed to be safe and comfortable.

The combination of breath and movement improves the meditation experience, taking practitioners to a state of deep stillness.

This holistic approach to well-being considers not just the physical elements of aging, but also the mental and emotional factors.

Chair yoga transforms into a haven for elders seeking peace and calm. The therapeutic effects go beyond the physical world, providing relief from the strains of everyday life.

As seniors immerse themselves in the seated yoga experience, they discover a tranquil realm in which the combination of breath and movement transforms into a source of vigor and calm.

The path of embracing calm via sitting yoga postures is a peaceful adventure for seniors over the age of 60.

Chair yoga provides a portal to a more peaceful living, promoting holistic well-being that extends beyond the boundaries of conventional practices.

Seniors may build a sense of calmness via the steady rhythm of sitting postures, which uplifts the soul, feeds the body, and provides a profound sense of quiet in their golden years.

Limbering Up: Chair-Based Gentle Stretches

Limbering up with chair-based easy stretches is a refreshing activity for seniors over 60, offering a comprehensive approach to physical well-being.

This chair-based yoga sequence is a moderate introduction to movement that promotes flexibility and increases general mobility.

Seniors can sit comfortably in a chair and perform a sequence of fluid stretches that target different muscle areas. These activities are intended to increase joint flexibility and alleviate stiffness that may accompany aging.

Participants engage in a low-impact workout tailored to their skills by including controlled twists, side bends, and forward folds.

The emphasis on attentive breathing during these chair stretches enhances their benefits. Deep, deliberate breathing promotes relaxation, lowers tension, and increases oxygen flow throughout the body.

This mindful breathing component adds to general well-being by encouraging a mind-body connection, which is critical for seniors.

Chair-based stretches for seniors, like any other exercise regimen, should be approached safely. The sitting posture gives a solid foundation, reducing the chance of falling or straining. This technique of limbering up is available to people of all abilities thanks to gentle movements and appropriate posture.

This chair yoga technique is both physically healthy and socially enjoyable. Group sessions allow elders to engage with others, creating a sense of community and support.

The shared experience of mild stretches in a chair fosters a good environment, making the exercise more pleasurable and motivating for participants.

Limbering up with chair-based easy stretches is an important addition to the wellness repertoire for seniors over 60.

It effortlessly combines exercise, breath, and community to promote physical and mental vigor in a safe and accessible setting.

Harmonizing Breath and Movement in Seated Postures

The integration of breath and movement is central to mindful movement practices designed for seniors, particularly in the setting of seated postures within chair yoga.

This specific type of yoga is designed for those over the age of 60, and it combines mild stretches with regulated breathing techniques.

Seated postures in chair yoga embody the notion of synchronicity, in which the ebb and flow of breath effortlessly integrate with intentional motions.

Seniors find comfort in the support of a chair, which allows for a progressive exploration of mobility and balance. As breath becomes the driving force, inhales and exhales serve as the tempo for each purposeful movement.

The mild undulations of the spine, twists, and side bends are accompanied by the rhythmic cadence of breathing.

This dance of breath and movement not only improves physical well-being, but it also builds a stronger connection to the moment.

This connection offers elders a route to improved body awareness and a sensation of tranquility, which promotes mental clarity.

Chair yoga for elders promotes accessibility, making it an inclusive practice for those with different levels of mobility. The combination of breath and movement promotes improved circulation, flexibility, and joint health. Furthermore, it creates a calm space for elders to practice mindfulness, which reduces stress and promotes emotional well-being.

The seamless integration of breath and movement in seated postures in chair yoga goes beyond the physical, harmonizing with the spiritual and mental levels.

It becomes a therapeutic trip for elders, with the chair serving as a vessel for holistic restoration.

Seniors elegantly negotiate these synchronized sequences, embarking on a journey that nurtures both body and soul, resulting in a symphony of well-being in their golden years.

Chapter 4: Chair-Based Meditation Practices

Chair-based meditation activities are a pleasant and accessible method for people over 60 to improve their overall health.

These practices include mindfulness within the framework of chair yoga, creating a sitting, comfortable environment for individuals to build inner calm and mental clarity.

Deep breathing exercises are an essential component of chair-based meditation in the context of chair yoga for elders.

This mindful breathing technique helps users center themselves in the present moment, which promotes relaxation and reduces tension. Seniors may safely engage in these contemplative breathing practices thanks to the supporting nature of sitting postures, which promotes a sense of serenity and contentment.

Furthermore, chair-based meditation approaches sometimes include guided imagery sessions.

Seniors are urged to envision peaceful landscapes or pleasant recollections via verbal cues, resulting in a mental escape within the limits of their chairs.

This not only improves the meditation experience but also leads to a more optimistic outlook and emotional well-being.

Chair yoga for elders focuses on gentle exercises that promote flexibility and mobility. These motions, along with focused awareness, result in an integrated meditation experience.

Seniors can investigate the delicate link between body and mind, cultivating peace and self-awareness.

Chair-based meditation techniques are adaptable to a wide range of physical abilities, making them an accessible alternative for seniors with various mobility capabilities.

This accessibility guarantees that those over 60 may meditate comfortably, generating feelings of empowerment and inclusiveness.

As part of chair yoga for seniors over 60, chair-based meditation activities provide a comprehensive approach to well-being.

By seamlessly blending breathwork, guided imagery, and mild exercises, these practices invite elders to embark on a journey of self-discovery, promoting both physical and mental vigor.

Cultivating Presence: Mindfulness in Seated Meditation

In the field of mindful practices for seniors over 60, cultivating presence via sitting meditation, particularly in the setting of chair yoga, has been shown to be a transforming activity.

This subtle yet deep method opens the door to improved well-being and overall health.

Seated meditation gives elders a unique opportunity to practice awareness while sitting comfortably in a chair. The key is to cultivate a high level of awareness and a strong connection between mind and body.

Individuals may practice mindfulness in this calm location without having to perform complex yoga positions.

The use of chair yoga in this contemplative journey meets the unique requirements of elders. The sitting posture offers stability, allowing people to engage comfortably regardless of their physical condition.

As elders focus on their breathing and internal feelings, the chair acts as a supporting anchor, providing a sense of security and relaxation.

The technique entails focusing attention on the current moment and gently correcting stray thoughts.

Seniors learn that the chair is more than a physical support; it is a symbolic bridge to a deeper connection with oneself. In this meditative zone, students learn to accept sensations without judgment, developing self-compassion.

The advantages continue beyond the current session, favorably altering daily living. Seniors increase their resilience to stress, improve their cognitive skills, and experience better emotional health.

Furthermore, the practice's simplicity makes it accessible to people of all fitness levels, which promotes inclusion.

The combination of sitting meditation and chair yoga creates a healthy partnership for elders seeking serenity. This practice not only fosters a profound feeling of presence, but it also teaches people to appreciate the beauty of the present moment, fostering a life of peace and contentment.

Serenity in Stillness: Guided Chair Meditation

Discover the serene realm of tranquility with guided chair meditation, designed exclusively for elders 60 and older.

Embracing the essence of silence, this one-of-a-kind practice blends chair yoga advantages with meditation aspects, resulting in a harmonic environment for mind and body alignment.

Seniors find comfort in the soft embrace of a chair as they go on a journey of inner peace. The guided meditation gradually guides people into mindfulness, encouraging mental clarity and emotional balance.

Individuals may easily achieve the peace that comes with a concentrated, meditative state while sitting in the chair's supporting construction.

The sitting posture provides a comfortable base, allowing elders to easily engage in deep breathing exercises.

Each breath serves as a channel for relaxation, cultivating a sense of calm that transcends the physical limitations of aging. Individuals may revitalize both their bodies and minds by engaging in focused breathing exercises.

As the guided meditation proceeds, participants are urged to relax and enjoy the present moment. The chair becomes a conduit for contemplation; its constant presence anchoring people in the present.

This focused connection with one's environment instills a sense of quiet that lasts beyond the meditation session, fostering long-term calm in daily life.

Chair meditation for elders over 60 demonstrates the versatility of health practices. It makes it possible for people to experience the deep advantages of meditation, which promote both physical relaxation and mental resilience.

Seniors find a haven in the silence of the guided practice, with the chair serving as a conduit to tranquility and each breath a soothing reminder of the serene path inside.

Elevating Mental Clarity through Breath Awareness

Chair yoga provides a unique opportunity for elders over 60 to improve mental clarity via breath awareness.

This mild type of exercise combines the advantages of yoga with the convenience of utilizing a chair, making it suitable for people who have restricted mobility.

Focusing on breath awareness becomes a key component, acting as a catalyst for improving mental health.

The practice includes conscious breathing methods that synchronize breath with movement. Seniors practice deep, deliberate inhalation and exhalation, which promotes heightened awareness.

This conscious link between breath and body movements increases oxygen flow, which improves circulation and cognitive function.

As a consequence, mental clarity improves, giving elders a practical opportunity to hone their cognitive skills.

Furthermore, chair yoga's focus on breathing helps to reduce tension. Seniors learn to release stress by taking regulated breaths, resulting in a calm and focused frame of mind.

This element is especially advantageous for seniors dealing with the problems of aging, since stress reduction has been related to increased cognitive performance and emotional wellbeing.

Chair yoga's simplicity makes it a viable alternative for seniors looking for mental clarity.

The integration of breath awareness is consistent with mindfulness ideals, allowing people to be completely present in the moment.

This mindfulness practice, combined with the physical advantages of chair yoga, provides a comprehensive approach to mental health.

In essence, chair yoga offers seniors over 60 a mild yet effective method of improving mental clarity.

By stressing breath awareness, this exercise transforms into a mindful journey that not only enhances cognitive performance but also develops a sense of calm, therefore boosting seniors' general mental health as they enter their golden years.

Chapter 5: Personalizing Your Chair Yoga Routine

Creating a personalized chair yoga regimen for seniors over 60 requires careful consideration of individual needs and preferences.

Personalization is essential to making the practice pleasurable, successful, and accessible to all participants.

 Begin by learning the individuals' distinct physical abilities and limits. Customize the routine to meet their unique needs, creating a sense of ease and empowerment.

Practice a variety of motions to improve flexibility, strength, and balance. Use mild stretches to increase mobility and reduce stiffness. Choose postures that cater to varying levels of flexibility, allowing individuals to advance at their own rate. This technique promotes a pleasurable experience and encourages consistent practice.

Mindful breathing is an essential component of chair yoga, facilitating relaxation and stress reduction. Incorporate breathing exercises effortlessly into your regimen to improve the mind-body connection.

Encourage participants to breathe deeply and rhythmically to promote a state of serenity and well-being.

To add a personal touch, consider including preferred music or calming noises that the participants enjoy. This not only creates a lovely environment but also makes the practice more pleasurable and interesting. Pay attention to any input and alter the program accordingly to fit individual needs.

To make sitting positions more comfortable, use props like cushions or blankets. This little change may make a big impact in assisting participants with various comfort levels and physical problems.

Personalized adaptations guarantee that every participant feels supported and capable during the session.

Keep open contact with participants, encouraging them to share their experiences and any obstacles they may encounter. Adapt the program depending on their comments to continually improve and customize the chair yoga experience.

By adapting the practice to individual requirements, chair yoga provides a balanced and pleasurable approach for seniors to improve their physical and mental health.

Tailoring the Practice: Customized Sequences

Adapting yoga practices to meet the unique requirements of seniors over 60, particularly those participating in chair yoga, entails adjusting sequences for maximum benefit.

Creating unique sequences for this group offers a thoughtful approach that takes into account their physical limits, flexibility, and general well-being.

Chair yoga postures are adapted to suit limited mobility and joint flexibility. A customized sequence might begin with easy warm-up activities that promote joint mobility and improve blood circulation.

These basic moves are intended to ease seniors into the practice and prepare their bodies for more difficult poses.

Seniors can focus on sitting positions that improve balance.

Stretches that target core strength and stability can assist improve posture and avoid falls. Breathing exercises are also effortlessly weaved throughout the routine, which promotes calm and attention.

Deep, regulated breathing not only promotes relaxation but also increases lung capacity and respiratory health.

A personalized chair yoga routine relies heavily on variety. Including a variety of activities ensures that different muscle groups are worked, increasing overall strength and flexibility. Customization enables teachers to choose poses that address specific issues in the elderly population, such as arthritis or back discomfort.

The speed of the practice should be moderate and careful, taking into account each participant's specific demands. Modifications should be encouraged, allowing elderly to alter positions to their comfort level.

This tailored approach creates a joyful and welcoming environment, allowing elderly to appreciate the practice without feeling forced or overwhelmed.

Tailoring chair yoga sequences for seniors over 60 involves more than just physical poses; it is a comprehensive strategy that takes into account their mental and emotional well-being. Integrating meditation or guided relaxation techniques into the practice promotes inner calm and awareness, which contributes to this lively demographic's overall well-being.

Chair yoga is an accessible and pleasurable trip for seniors, boosting health and energy in their golden years thanks to customized sequences that have been carefully created.m

Adapting Asanas: Variations for Diverse Abilities

Embracing inclusion in yoga entails customizing practices to meet various abilities, making it accessible to all. Chair yoga is a mild yet effective modification for seniors over the age of 60. This modified technique enables anyone with various physical capacities to get the many benefits of yoga without the requirement for standard floor positions.

Chair yoga provides a solid foundation for elders by encouraging balance, flexibility, and relaxation. Begin in a sitting mountain position, anchoring people by connecting with the chair. Move into mild twists to improve spine mobility and digestion.

The chair becomes a prop for modified standing postures, allowing for strength development without the strain of full weight-bearing workouts.

Sun salutations can be modified with sitting versions to improve circulation and energy.

Encouraging mild upper-body motions, such as arm stretches and neck rotations, reduces stress and increases joint flexibility. Breathwork is essential for cultivating awareness and relaxation.

Chair aerobics may be used to increase heart rate without jeopardizing safety.

Balancing postures, such as tree pose, may be performed using the chair for support, offering a sense of success and increased stability.

Adapting asanas for different capacities goes beyond the physical considerations. Meditation and visualization exercises improve mental well-being.

Guided relaxation in the chair allows elders to decompress, reducing tension and improving sleep quality.

Chair yoga for elders over 60 demonstrates the versatility of this ancient technique.

Individuals of all capacities may get the comprehensive advantages of yoga by embracing variations and changes.

This method promotes not just physical well-being but also mental and emotional wellness, making yoga a welcoming and fulfilling practice for everybody.

Personal Empowerment: Chair Yoga for Individual Needs

Personal empowerment via chair yoga is a revolutionary experience, particularly for seniors aged 60 and over.

 This gentle practice addresses individual requirements, promoting physical well-being, mental clarity, and emotional harmony.

Chair yoga provides a unique approach to health, making it accessible to seniors of varying physical capacities.

This empowering practice transforms classic yoga postures into sitting or supported positions, creating a safe and welcoming setting.

Regardless of their present fitness level, participants increase their flexibility, strength, and balance.

Beyond the physical advantages, chair yoga may be used to promote mindfulness and reduce stress.

Seniors do breathing exercises and meditation to promote mental clarity and relaxation.

This all-encompassing method not only improves cognitive performance but also enables people to face life's problems with a renewed feeling of serenity and resilience.

One of the most impressive qualities of chair yoga is its capacity to adapt to individual requirements. In a supportive group context, seniors can modify the practice to address individual issues, such as joint stiffness, limited mobility, or chronic diseases.

This tailored approach promotes a sense of agency and control over one's well-being, allowing elderly to actively engage in their health journey.

Chair yoga acts as a social outlet, fostering a sense of belonging among participants.

The shared experience of growth and self-discovery improves interpersonal relationships, reducing feelings of loneliness.

This sense of belonging helps to empower elders by reaffirming their importance and contribution in the community.

Chair yoga is emerging as a significant tool for seniors' personal empowerment. This technique goes beyond standard workout regimens since it addresses individual requirements while also establishing a supportive community.

Seniors over 60 discover a road to comprehensive well-being by incorporating physical vitality, mental resilience, and a profound feeling of empowerment into their everyday lives.

Chapter 6: Safety Measures and Precautions

It is critical to ensure the safety of seniors over the age of 60 who practice chair yoga.

As people age, their bodies may lose flexibility and balance; thus, it is critical to employ adequate safety precautions during these sessions.

To begin, pick a solid and stable chair to reduce the danger of falls or accidents. Opting for a chair with a straight back and no wheels improves overall stability during yoga practice.

Furthermore, elders should be urged to choose comfortable attire that does not limit movement, promotes ease, and avoids pain. The significance of excellent posture cannot be overstated, since keeping a neutral spine aligns the body and reduces joint strain.

Gentle reminders to participants to listen to their bodies and avoid pushing themselves beyond their comfort zones help to ensure a safe and pleasurable experience.

Chair yoga safety relies heavily on instructor direction. Instructors must offer clear and succinct verbal signals to aid comprehension and reduce the likelihood of improper movements.

A progressive development through poses allows seniors to adapt at their own rate, reducing the risk of injury. It is critical for teachers to be sensitive to their students' particular requirements, making adjustments as needed to accommodate varied degrees of mobility.

Proper warm-up activities are required before attempting more complicated positions.

Gentle exercises that promote blood flow and flexibility prepare the body for the yoga practice, lowering the risk of strains and injuries.

Hydration is another important factor that is often ignored; seniors should be encouraged to remain hydrated during the session.

Prioritizing safety measures and precautions in chair yoga for seniors over 60 requires careful consideration of chair selection, clothes, posture, teacher direction, progressive progression, warm-up activities, and hydration. By following these instructions, seniors may enjoy the physical and emotional advantages of chair yoga without jeopardizing their health.

Ensuring Secure Practice Spaces for Seniors

Creating safe practice environments for seniors who participate in chair yoga is critical for their health and the pleasure of the exercise.

Safety should be a key concern, with the goal of keeping the environment free of any threats.

Adequate illumination is critical to preventing trips and falls and instilling a sense of security while practicing.

Furthermore, installing non-slip mats beneath the seats adds stability and reduces the danger of accidents.

Furthermore, instructors must adjust their courses to the diverse fitness levels and physical problems of elders. Offering adapted postures and gentle motions ensures that people of all capacities can participate safely.

This openness fosters a supportive environment, creating a sense of community among participants.

Instructors should also be knowledgeable of senior health issues, keeping participants informed of any medical illnesses or physical restrictions they may have.

This understanding allows them to give personalized coaching, ensuring that each senior can practice chair yoga with confidence and ease.

Regular communication with participants about their health and any issues they may have is essential for building a safe and supportive environment.

Introducing mindfulness into chair yoga sessions can help to create a safe practice atmosphere.

Encouraging seniors to focus on their breath and be present in the moment not only improves the mental advantages of the exercise, but also minimizes the possibility of distractions that might lead to an accident.

Overall, maintaining safe practice spaces for seniors doing chair yoga necessitates a comprehensive strategy that considers physical, emotional, and environmental factors.

Instructors may create an environment in which elders can confidently and enjoyably accept the advantages of chair yoga by focusing on safety, inclusivity, and customized assistance.

Proactive Health Measures in Chair Yoga

Ensuring the well-being of seniors over 60 with chair yoga entails implementing preventive health measures tailored to their specific needs.

Gentle motions and stretches done while seated in a chair can help improve flexibility, balance, and general physical health.

Chair yoga for seniors involves attentive breathing techniques that promote relaxation and stress reduction. These activities not only promote mental health but also help to improve respiratory function.

Chair yoga's regulated breathing helps seniors manage anxiety and increase their emotional resilience.

The sitting poses in chair yoga are designed to improve joint mobility, particularly in regions that tend to stiffen as we age.

Chair yoga helps seniors avoid pain and improves their ability to do everyday tasks by fostering a wide range of motion. Regular practice also promotes improved circulation, which is essential for preserving cardiovascular health.

Balance is a major problem for seniors, and chair yoga addresses this by including stability exercises. These chair-supported exercises provide a safe setting for elders to improve their balance and minimize the chance of falling.

This component is very useful in fostering independence and confidence in daily movements.

Chair yoga stresses mindfulness and relaxation practices to promote mental clarity and emotional well-being.

Seniors feel calm as they join in the gradual flow of exercises, which promotes a good outlook and reduces stress.

Preventative health measures in chair yoga for seniors over 60 use a holistic approach. The personalized practice fosters a better, more balanced lifestyle, including joint flexibility, respiratory health, and mental well-being.

Integrating chair yoga into a daily practice enables seniors to manage their health more effectively and have a higher quality of life.

Demystifying Concerns: Chair Yoga Safety Insights

Investigating the safety concerns of chair yoga for seniors over the age of 60 reveals a more sophisticated approach to overall well-being.

As people age, maintaining flexibility and strength becomes increasingly important for their general health.

Chair yoga is a gentle yet effective method of reaching these aims, suited particularly to the specialized requirements of elders.

To begin, the use of adaptable movements in chair yoga guarantees that elders may exercise without excessive strain.

The emphasis on fluidity and smooth transitions reduces the danger of injury, making it an excellent exercise for people with mobility issues.

Participants may comfortably complete postures while using a chair as support, developing a sense of security and confidence.

Furthermore, chair yoga promotes awareness, mental clarity, and relaxation. As seniors handle life's complications, incorporating breathwork and meditation into chair yoga sessions provides a therapeutic outlet for stress reduction.

This not only improves mental well-being, but it also benefits physical health by lowering stress and increasing sleep quality.

Providing a safe chair yoga experience requires personalized training from qualified instructors.

Professionals who are skilled in adapting poses to suit different abilities and health problems play an important part in creating a supportive atmosphere.

Seniors benefit from customized supervision, which allows them to approach the practice at their own speed and comfort level.

It is critical to acknowledge the inclusive aspect of chair yoga, which makes it accessible to everyone with a variety of physical capabilities.

By dispelling myths about chair yoga, seniors may embrace this fascinating practice, opening the door to greater flexibility, strength, and overall health. By carefully addressing safety concerns, chair yoga develops not just as a fitness regimen, but also as a comprehensive strategy to fostering well-being in the golden years.

Chapter 7: Beyond the Chair: Integrating Yoga Into Daily Life

In the field of holistic well-being, adding yoga outside of a typical practice space has proven to be a transforming strategy, particularly for seniors aged 60 and over.

Beyond the chair, yoga blends into everyday life, providing several advantages for physical health, cerebral clarity, and emotional balance.

For elders, chair yoga is a gentle yet effective way to improve flexibility, balance, and overall mobility.

Yoga positions are adaptable to a sitting position, making them accessible to people who may struggle with typical floor exercises. Seniors can develop strength and resilience by incorporating chair-based techniques into their daily routines, encouraging a sense of independence.

Furthermore, the contemplative features of yoga considerably improve mental health. Mindful breathing exercises not only improve lung capacity but also help to reduce stress.

 Seniors may easily include moments of mindfulness into their daily routine, whether they are sitting at a desk or drinking tea.
 This thoughtful approach to regular tasks improves cognitive performance and fosters a state of serenity.

Embracing yoga beyond the mat entails adopting a yogic mentality in everyday encounters. Compassion, appreciation, and self-awareness may be integrated into talks and interactions to promote a peaceful and happy social life.

Seniors who incorporate these ideals into their everyday lives might feel a strong sense of connection and purpose.

In essence, the incorporation of yoga into daily life extends beyond the physical components of practice.

It becomes a mindset that pervades one's entire life, supporting overall well-being for seniors entering their golden years.

Beyond the chair, yoga becomes a guiding force, instilling perseverance, serenity, and a revitalized enthusiasm for living.

Transcending Boundaries: Applying Chair Yoga Beyond Sessions

Chair yoga for seniors over 60 provides a transforming experience that goes far beyond the scope of typical sessions.

Embracing the essence of transcendence, this practice evolves into a comprehensive journey that promotes physical, mental, and emotional wellness.

Beyond the chair and mat, its influence extends throughout everyday life, breaking down barriers and smoothly blending into routine tasks.

The beauty of chair yoga is its versatility, which makes it a useful companion outside of official sessions. Seniors readily incorporate attentive movements into their everyday activities, bringing moments of quiet into the commonplace. As they sit comfortably, the practice expands into the domains of flexibility, balance, and strength, improving mobility in surprising ways.

Beyond the physical, chair yoga promotes mental clarity and emotional resilience.

The breathwork, a cornerstone of this practice, extends beyond the constraints of a yoga class and becomes a tool for stress management in a variety of settings.

Seniors use the power of mindful breathing to create a pocket of peace in the middle of life's pressures, whether they're waiting in line or sitting down to eat.

Chair yoga also breaks down social barriers, encouraging elderly to feel more connected.

Shared experiences throughout sessions foster long-term ties that transcend beyond the yoga studio.

Seniors help one other by sharing ideas and encouragement, resulting in a network that improves the fabric of their everyday lives.

Chair yoga bridges cultural and generational differences. As its ideals infiltrate seniors' everyday routines, younger generations grow intrigued and amenable to adopting these thoughtful habits.

The intergenerational flow of wisdom becomes a natural byproduct, reducing preconceptions and boosting understanding.

Chair yoga for seniors over 60 goes beyond the concept of a planned program.

It evolves into a dynamic force that pervades all aspects of life, encouraging bodily well-being, mental clarity, social connection, and intergenerational understanding.

Its influence is felt not just on the mat, but also in the seamless integration of mindful moments into the fabric of everyday life.

Radiant Living: Chair Yoga's Holistic Impact

Radiant Living recognizes the tremendous advantages of chair yoga for elders 60 and above, promoting a comprehensive approach to well-being.

This easy kind of exercise improves physical, mental, and emotional wellbeing without requiring difficult positions. Individuals benefit from greater flexibility, balance, and mobility.

In terms of physical well-being, chair yoga provides a low-impact option that is accessible to seniors of all fitness levels.

The mild stretches and motions help to relieve stiffness, reduce joint soreness, and improve general flexibility. This not only benefits physical health but also promotes independence and vigor.

Beyond the physical domain, chair yoga has a comprehensive influence on the mind and emotions.

The technique promotes attention and relaxation, creating a peaceful mental environment for elders.

It acts as a therapeutic tool, reducing tension and encouraging a positive outlook. Individuals who participate in the rhythmic flow of chair yoga enjoy a sense of calm that spreads throughout their everyday life.

Furthermore, chair yoga is a social activity that promotes seniors' emotional well-being. Group sessions establish a friendly environment by encouraging relationships and a sense of camaraderie. This social dimension is essential to holistic living because it covers a larger range of human needs beyond just physical activity.

In essence, Radiant Living's approach to chair yoga for seniors over 60 demonstrates the linked nature of well-being.

Chair yoga illuminates a bright and meaningful existence by smoothly combining physical, mental, and emotional components.

Individuals who start on this comprehensive journey experience not only improved physical vigor but also a profound sense of tranquility and connection.

Sustaining Well-being: Chair Yoga Principles in Daily Practices

Sustaining well-being is an important part of living a satisfying life, especially for seniors over 60 who may have physical restrictions.

Chair yoga is a gentle yet effective technique to enhance health and vitality without the need for a yoga mat or hard motions.

Using chair yoga concepts in everyday practice creates a comprehensive approach to promoting overall wellbeing.

Breath awareness is a crucial aspect of chair yoga. Seniors are recommended to practice deep, purposeful breathing to increase lung capacity and oxygenate the body.

This awareness not only helps lung health, but it also lowers stress and increases mental clarity.

Chair yoga regimens rely heavily on balancing postures. Seniors should exercise mild weight shifting and controlled movements while seated to improve stability and prevent falls.

These exercises help to increase coordination and physical strength, which are vital for retaining independence as we age.

Chair yoga also emphasizes flexibility. Gentle stretches can improve joint mobility and minimize stiffness. Seniors can gradually expand their range of motion, improving circulation and lowering the risk of joint pain.

Chair yoga emphasizes the mind-body connection, which promotes calm. Seniors can reduce anxiety and improve their mental health by practicing meditation and mindfulness practices.

This holistic approach recognizes the interdependence of physical and mental health, which contributes to a sense of balance.

Chair yoga is adjustable, making it suitable for seniors of various capacities. Individual requirements may be accommodated through modifications, resulting in a safe and inclusive practice for all.

Seniors who incorporate chair yoga concepts into their daily routines can experience increased physical health, emotional well-being, and a renewed feeling of vigor, eventually preserving their entire well-being in a thoughtful and joyful way.

CONCLUSION

Chair yoga provides a comprehensive and accessible method for enhancing the physical, mental, and emotional well-being of seniors over the age of sixty.

Chair yoga, which adapts basic yoga postures to sitting positions, delivers several advantages tailored particularly to the requirements and constraints of older people.

Physically, chair yoga improves seniors' flexibility, strength, balance, and posture. Seniors can relieve stiffness, minimize joint discomfort, and enhance their range of motion by stretching and moving gently while seated.

Chair yoga improves circulation and cardiovascular health, boosting overall physical vigor and resilience.

Mentally, chair yoga promotes attention and relaxation, which helps elders manage stress, anxiety, and depression. The emphasis on regulated breathing methods fosters a sense of quiet and tranquility, improving mental clarity and emotional well-being.

Furthermore, chair yoga promotes self-awareness and acceptance, allowing seniors to appreciate their bodies and skills with compassion and optimism.

Socially, chair yoga offers seniors a friendly and inclusive environment in which to interact with others, share experiences, and form meaningful connections. Group chair yoga classes provide chances for social engagement and companionship, which helps to reduce feelings of isolation and loneliness that many older persons suffer.

Chair yoga is adaptive and customizable, making it appropriate for seniors with varying fitness levels and physical limitations.

 Chair yoga may be adapted to individual requirements and preferences, whether you're recuperating from an accident, managing chronic diseases, or simply want to maintain your general health and vitality.

Chair yoga is a vital and accessible health activity for seniors over 60, with several physical, emotional, and social advantages.

By introducing chair yoga into their daily routine, older individuals may improve their quality of life, promote healthy aging, and build a sense of well-being that goes beyond the yoga mat.

Workout Planner for Seniors

	EXERCISE	GOAL
MON DAY		
TUES DAY		
WEDNES DAY		
THURS DAY		
FRI DAY		
SAT DAY		

Workout Planner
for Seniors

	EXERCISE	GOAL
MON DAY		
TUES DAY		
WEDNES DAY		
THURS DAY		
FRI DAY		
SAT DAY		

Workout Planner for Seniors

	EXERCISE	GOAL
MON DAY		
TUES DAY		
WEDNES DAY		
THURS DAY		
FRI DAY		
SAT DAY		

Workout Planner for Seniors

	EXERCISE	GOAL
MON DAY		
TUES DAY		
WEDNES DAY		
THURS DAY		
FRI DAY		
SAT DAY		

Workout Planner for Seniors

	EXERCISE	GOAL
MON DAY		
TUES DAY		
WEDNES DAY		
THURS DAY		
FRI DAY		
SAT DAY		

Workout Planner for Seniors

	EXERCISE	GOAL
MON DAY		
TUES DAY		
WEDNES DAY		
THURS DAY		
FRI DAY		
SAT DAY		

Workout Planner for Seniors

	EXERCISE	GOAL
MON DAY		
TUES DAY		
WEDNES DAY		
THURS DAY		
FRI DAY		
SAT DAY		

Workout Planner for Seniors

	EXERCISE	GOAL
MON DAY		
TUES DAY		
WEDNES DAY		
THURS DAY		
FRI DAY		
SAT DAY		

Workout Planner
for Seniors

	EXERCISE	GOAL
MON DAY		
TUES DAY		
WEDNES DAY		
THURS DAY		
FRI DAY		
SAT DAY		

Workout Planner
for Seniors

	EXERCISE	GOAL
MON DAY		
TUES DAY		
WEDNES DAY		
THURS DAY		
FRI DAY		
SAT DAY		

Workout Planner for Seniors

	EXERCISE	GOAL
MON DAY		
TUES DAY		
WEDNES DAY		
THURS DAY		
FRI DAY		
SAT DAY		

Workout Planner
for Seniors

	EXERCISE	GOAL
MON DAY		
TUES DAY		
WEDNES DAY		
THURS DAY		
FRI DAY		
SAT DAY		

Workout Planner for Seniors

	EXERCISE	GOAL
MON DAY		
TUES DAY		
WEDNES DAY		
THURS DAY		
FRI DAY		
SAT DAY		

Workout Planner for Seniors

	EXERCISE	GOAL
MON DAY		
TUES DAY		
WEDNES DAY		
THURS DAY		
FRI DAY		
SAT DAY		

Workout Planner for Seniors

	EXERCISE	GOAL
MON DAY		
TUES DAY		
WEDNES DAY		
THURS DAY		
FRI DAY		
SAT DAY		

Workout Planner for Seniors

	EXERCISE	GOAL
MON DAY		
TUES DAY		
WEDNES DAY		
THURS DAY		
FRI DAY		
SAT DAY		

Workout Planner for Seniors

	EXERCISE	GOAL
MON DAY		
TUES DAY		
WEDNES DAY		
THURS DAY		
FRI DAY		
SAT DAY		

Workout Planner for Seniors

	EXERCISE	GOAL
MON DAY		
TUES DAY		
WEDNES DAY		
THURS DAY		
FRI DAY		
SAT DAY		

Workout Planner for Seniors

	EXERCISE	GOAL
MON DAY		
TUES DAY		
WEDNES DAY		
THURS DAY		
FRI DAY		
SAT DAY		

Workout Planner for Seniors

	EXERCISE	GOAL
MON DAY		
TUES DAY		
WEDNES DAY		
THURS DAY		
FRI DAY		
SAT DAY		

Workout Planner for Seniors

	EXERCISE	GOAL
MON DAY		
TUES DAY		
WEDNES DAY		
THURS DAY		
FRI DAY		
SAT DAY		

Workout Planner for Seniors

	EXERCISE	GOAL
MON DAY		
TUES DAY		
WEDNES DAY		
THURS DAY		
FRI DAY		
SAT DAY		

Workout Planner for Seniors

	EXERCISE	GOAL
MON DAY		
TUES DAY		
WEDNES DAY		
THURS DAY		
FRI DAY		
SAT DAY		

139

Workout Planner for Seniors

	EXERCISE	GOAL
MON DAY		
TUES DAY		
WEDNES DAY		
THURS DAY		
FRI DAY		
SAT DAY		

Workout Planner for Seniors

	EXERCISE	GOAL
MON DAY		
TUES DAY		
WEDNES DAY		
THURS DAY		
FRI DAY		
SAT DAY		

Workout Planner for Seniors

	EXERCISE	GOAL
MON DAY		
TUES DAY		
WEDNES DAY		
THURS DAY		
FRI DAY		
SAT DAY		

Workout Planner
for Seniors

	EXERCISE	GOAL
MON DAY		
TUES DAY		
WEDNES DAY		
THURS DAY		
FRI DAY		
SAT DAY		

Workout Planner for Seniors

	EXERCISE	GOAL
MON DAY		
TUES DAY		
WEDNES DAY		
THURS DAY		
FRI DAY		
SAT DAY		

Workout Planner for Seniors

	EXERCISE	GOAL
MON DAY		
TUES DAY		
WEDNES DAY		
THURS DAY		
FRI DAY		
SAT DAY		

Workout Planner for Seniors

	EXERCISE	GOAL
MON DAY		
TUES DAY		
WEDNES DAY		
THURS DAY		
FRI DAY		
SAT DAY		

Workout Planner for Seniors

	EXERCISE	GOAL
MON DAY		
TUES DAY		
WEDNES DAY		
THURS DAY		
FRI DAY		
SAT DAY		

Workout Planner for Seniors

	EXERCISE	GOAL
MON DAY		
TUES DAY		
WEDNES DAY		
THURS DAY		
FRI DAY		
SAT DAY		

Workout Planner
for Seniors

	EXERCISE	GOAL
MON DAY		
TUES DAY		
WEDNES DAY		
THURS DAY		
FRI DAY		
SAT DAY		

Workout Planner for Seniors

	EXERCISE	GOAL
MON DAY		
TUES DAY		
WEDNES DAY		
THURS DAY		
FRI DAY		
SAT DAY		

Workout Planner for Seniors

	EXERCISE	GOAL
MON DAY		
TUES DAY		
WEDNES DAY		
THURS DAY		
FRI DAY		
SAT DAY		

Workout Planner for Seniors

	EXERCISE	GOAL
MON DAY		
TUES DAY		
WEDNES DAY		
THURS DAY		
FRI DAY		
SAT DAY		

Workout Planner for Seniors

	EXERCISE	GOAL
MON DAY		
TUES DAY		
WEDNES DAY		
THURS DAY		
FRI DAY		
SAT DAY		

Workout Planner
for Seniors

	EXERCISE	GOAL
MON DAY		
TUES DAY		
WEDNES DAY		
THURS DAY		
FRI DAY		
SAT DAY		

Workout Planner
for Seniors

	EXERCISE	GOAL
MON DAY		
TUES DAY		
WEDNES DAY		
THURS DAY		
FRI DAY		
SAT DAY		

Workout Planner
for Seniors

	EXERCISE	GOAL
MON DAY		
TUES DAY		
WEDNES DAY		
THURS DAY		
FRI DAY		
SAT DAY		

Workout Planner
for Seniors

	EXERCISE	GOAL
MON DAY		
TUES DAY		
WEDNES DAY		
THURS DAY		
FRI DAY		
SAT DAY		

Workout Planner for Seniors

	EXERCISE	GOAL
MON DAY		
TUES DAY		
WEDNES DAY		
THURS DAY		
FRI DAY		
SAT DAY		

Workout Planner for Seniors

	EXERCISE	GOAL
MON DAY		
TUES DAY		
WEDNES DAY		
THURS DAY		
FRI DAY		
SAT DAY		

Workout Planner for Seniors

	EXERCISE	GOAL
MON DAY		
TUES DAY		
WEDNES DAY		
THURS DAY		
FRI DAY		
SAT DAY		

Workout Planner for Seniors

	EXERCISE	GOAL
MON DAY		
TUES DAY		
WEDNES DAY		
THURS DAY		
FRI DAY		
SAT DAY		

Workout Planner for Seniors

	EXERCISE	GOAL
MON DAY		
TUES DAY		
WEDNES DAY		
THURS DAY		
FRI DAY		
SAT DAY		

Workout Planner for Seniors

	EXERCISE	GOAL
MON DAY		
TUES DAY		
WEDNES DAY		
THURS DAY		
FRI DAY		
SAT DAY		

Workout Planner for Seniors

	EXERCISE	GOAL
MON DAY		
TUES DAY		
WEDNES DAY		
THURS DAY		
FRI DAY		
SAT DAY		

Workout Planner for Seniors

	EXERCISE	GOAL
MON DAY		
TUES DAY		
WEDNES DAY		
THURS DAY		
FRI DAY		
SAT DAY		

Workout Planner
for Seniors

	EXERCISE	GOAL
MON DAY		
TUES DAY		
WEDNES DAY		
THURS DAY		
FRI DAY		
SAT DAY		

Workout Planner
for Seniors

	EXERCISE	GOAL
MON DAY		
TUES DAY		
WEDNES DAY		
THURS DAY		
FRI DAY		
SAT DAY		

Workout Planner for Seniors

	EXERCISE	GOAL
MON DAY		
TUES DAY		
WEDNES DAY		
THURS DAY		
FRI DAY		
SAT DAY		

Workout Planner for Seniors

	EXERCISE	GOAL
MON DAY		
TUES DAY		
WEDNES DAY		
THURS DAY		
FRI DAY		
SAT DAY		

Workout Planner for Seniors

	EXERCISE	GOAL
MON DAY		
TUES DAY		
WEDNES DAY		
THURS DAY		
FRI DAY		
SAT DAY		

Workout Planner for Seniors

	EXERCISE	GOAL
MON DAY		
TUES DAY		
WEDNES DAY		
THURS DAY		
FRI DAY		
SAT DAY		

Workout Planner for Seniors

	EXERCISE	GOAL
MON DAY		
TUES DAY		
WEDNES DAY		
THURS DAY		
FRI DAY		
SAT DAY		

Workout Planner for Seniors

	EXERCISE	GOAL
MON DAY		
TUES DAY		
WEDNES DAY		
THURS DAY		
FRI DAY		
SAT DAY		

Workout Planner for Seniors

	EXERCISE	GOAL
MON DAY		
TUES DAY		
WEDNES DAY		
THURS DAY		
FRI DAY		
SAT DAY		

Workout Planner
for Seniors

	EXERCISE	GOAL
MON DAY		
TUES DAY		
WEDNES DAY		
THURS DAY		
FRI DAY		
SAT DAY		

Workout Planner for Seniors

	EXERCISE	GOAL
MON DAY		
TUES DAY		
WEDNES DAY		
THURS DAY		
FRI DAY		
SAT DAY		

Workout Planner for Seniors

	EXERCISE	GOAL
MON DAY		
TUES DAY		
WEDNES DAY		
THURS DAY		
FRI DAY		
SAT DAY		

Workout Planner for Seniors

	EXERCISE	GOAL
MON DAY		
TUES DAY		
WEDNES DAY		
THURS DAY		
FRI DAY		
SAT DAY		

Workout Planner for Seniors

	EXERCISE	GOAL
MON DAY		
TUES DAY		
WEDNES DAY		
THURS DAY		
FRI DAY		
SAT DAY		

Workout Planner for Seniors

	EXERCISE	GOAL
MON DAY		
TUES DAY		
WEDNES DAY		
THURS DAY		
FRI DAY		
SAT DAY		

Workout Planner for Seniors

	EXERCISE	GOAL
MON DAY		
TUES DAY		
WEDNES DAY		
THURS DAY		
FRI DAY		
SAT DAY		

Workout Planner for Seniors

	EXERCISE	GOAL
MON DAY		
TUES DAY		
WEDNES DAY		
THURS DAY		
FRI DAY		
SAT DAY		

Workout Planner for Seniors

	EXERCISE	GOAL
MON DAY		
TUES DAY		
WEDNES DAY		
THURS DAY		
FRI DAY		
SAT DAY		

Workout Planner
for Seniors

	EXERCISE	GOAL
MON DAY		
TUES DAY		
WEDNES DAY		
THURS DAY		
FRI DAY		
SAT DAY		

Workout Planner for Seniors

	EXERCISE	GOAL
MON DAY		
TUES DAY		
WEDNES DAY		
THURS DAY		
FRI DAY		
SAT DAY		

Workout Planner for Seniors

	EXERCISE	GOAL
MON DAY		
TUES DAY		
WEDNES DAY		
THURS DAY		
FRI DAY		
SAT DAY		

Workout Planner for Seniors

	EXERCISE	GOAL
MON DAY		
TUES DAY		
WEDNES DAY		
THURS DAY		
FRI DAY		
SAT DAY		

Workout Planner for Seniors

	EXERCISE	GOAL
MON DAY		
TUES DAY		
WEDNES DAY		
THURS DAY		
FRI DAY		
SAT DAY		

Workout Planner for Seniors

	EXERCISE	GOAL
MON DAY		
TUES DAY		
WEDNES DAY		
THURS DAY		
FRI DAY		
SAT DAY